THE FIGHTING SPIRIT

THE ART OF WINNING YOUR FIGHT

BY **MARY McALARY**
AND **GEORGE FOREMAN III**

WITH ALICE SULLIVAN

CHANGING LIVES PRESS

This book contains advice and information related to healthcare. It is not intended to replace medical advice and should be used to supplement rather than replace regular care by your doctor. It is recommended that you seek your physician's advice before embarking on any health plan. The Publisher and the Author disclaim liability for any medical outcomes that may occur as a result of applying the methods suggested in this book.

Mention of specific companies, organizations, or authorities in this book does not imply endorsement by the Author or Publisher, nor does mention of specific companies, organizations, or authorities imply that they endorse this book, it's author, or the Publisher.

Internet addresses and telephone numbers given in this book were accurate at the time it went to press.

 CHANGING LIVES PRESS
P.O. Box 140189
Howard Beach, NY 11414
www.changinglivespress.com

Library of Congress Cataloging-in-Publication Data is available
through the Library of Congress.

Copyright © 2014 FC Brand, LLC

ISBN: 978-0-9904396-2-2

Printed in the United States of America

Written with Alice Sullivan, www.alicesullivan.com.

10 9 8 7 6 5 4 3 2 1

To anyone and everyone
who wants to give up but shouldn't,
who has hit rock bottom and
wants to come back swinging,
who is in pain, has heard bad
news from doctors' reports,
shed tears and yet wants to
emerge a stronger person,
THIS BOOK IS FOR YOU.

●

Mary McAlary and George Foreman III

CONTENTS

INTRODUCTION

by George Foreman III

FIGHTING WORDS

SUCCESS IS NOT DEFINED BY WINS OR LOSSES, but by the journey. That's not some cute, feel-good quote to stick on your refrigerator. It's the truth—both for my life and for yours. My story is not one of triumph, one of victory, or one of loss, but one of undying optimism that if you wake up every day and FIGHT, you can accomplish anything. This is what my father instilled in me, and this is the attitude I take into everything I do. Life has knocked me down a few times, but I've learned that it is not about the results but about the attitude and effort to be better. It's about chomping at the bit to wake up and defy the odds every day.

MY FIGHT

I exist to be an inspiration to empower as many people as possible with the education, tools, support, and attitude to get up and FIGHT for a better life, no matter what it takes. This required that I build a team of real fighters, TRUE FIGHTERS, who embody the EVERYBODY FIGHTS attitude and take it into everything they do, a team I can rely on to help me inspire and assist others to FIGHT for their health, happiness, and success at anything their heart desires, whether it's related to business, family, health, or redemption.

No one walks through this world alone. Even professional athletes have a group of individuals to work with them, encourage them, and challenge them to be the best at what they do. Likewise, if you want to overcome an illness, perform better, reach higher and more challenging goals, and make the most of each day, it's much easier to do when you have a team of Mary McAlary and friends cheering you on.

Regardless of the circumstances, if you want to achieve something positive, and you are willing and able to convince my team of your sincere burning desire to fight for it, we will support your fight by giving you tools such as the Fight Laws and the ability to share your story with our community. How? Join our EverybodyFights community, pay it forward with your story, and inspire others to share their stories and motivate our community of Everyday Fighters.

THE "EVERYBODYFIGHTS" COMMUNITY

My pilgrimage is to build a community of fighters that inspire through storytelling. Along my travels with my dad who has been a minister all my life. Over the years, he has transformed his life from being extremely poor to a boxing champion, father, a minister since 1977, and a businessman. I had the opportunity to meet many people from all walks of life. Their stories inspired me to want more from my life and to build a positive community for others. They also inspired me to start a professional boxing career and to leave it for something bigger three years later. Too much nowadays we are focused on the negative because that is what we are surrounded by: negativity and the inability to effect our own outcomes. What we need is to surround ourselves with EVERYDAY FIGHTERS and their stories. Everyday people that wake up and face life head on and see obstacles as challenges. Don't get me wrong; challenges are not fun and they do everything they can to get in the way of growth, happiness, and success. But I believe that with the right attitude, the right support network, and the right perspective, we can fight anything. . . . WHY? Because I have seen it firsthand and I will show those that may be skeptical that by fighting every day, you will reap benefits you never thought possible. It won't be easy and you will be pushed well beyond what you thought you were capable of, but happiness and contentment is possible if you fight. Those that fight together stay together. I hope you enjoy Mary's story and take with you the Fight Laws, Fight Facts, and everyday lessons to aid in your fight and efforts to win your everyday fight. I also hope you will join our community of fighters and let your fight story help others who are fighting just like you. Please join the fight community and share your story by interacting via Twitter and Instagram #WHYIFIGHT or sending us your story through our website www.thefightingspirit. com. Yours might be the next story profiled in our book series just like Mary's and serve as an inspiration for so many.

MARY'S FIGHT

Mary is the epitome of an Everyday Fighter. I met her while trying to learn the art of nutrition when I moved up to Boston to open my Gym and Lifestyle Fitness business. Mary, in her early 60s, walked in the room with a glow about her that I rarely see from any human being I have met. She had an aura and an energy that she not only carried with her but passed on to others. I instantly became enamored with her, and I just knew I needed to know her story. Little did I know that I would spend the next 16 months with her crafting this story, a story I carry with me to this day.

THE ART OF WINNING YOUR FIGHT

Mary McAlary was dealt a deck of cards that could not have been foreseen or prevented. She not only fights for her daily health, but for the health of others. Mary's goal is to enlighten and teach others how to do so. Living an unhealthy lifestyle should be a conscious decision, not an accident or something one has been tricked into. Mary's goal is to fight choreographed confusion created by profit-hungry corporations whose own employees won't even consume their own products. That alone should be enough to make you think twice about what fuel you choose to put into your body.

When it comes to making a life change, information is the first step; motivation and support to do better is the next. That's why I have chosen Mary to kick off the EVERYBODYFIGHTS book series. She fights every day for her own health, but more importantly, to Pay It Forward to build her community of Everyday Fighters . . . who fight to maintain their health. As a good friend, Jim Coghlin from 15-40 Connection (15-40.0rg), once told me:

"Health is wealth. For without it you have little."

Read Mary's story. Digest her wisdom. Get tattooed with inspiration as she tells her incredible story of beating the odds.

By the end of this story, I am confident you will join our community of Everyday Fighters, help us build the Fighting Spirit, and share your stories with us.

Fight on.

Sincerely,

George Edward "Monk" Foreman III

Fighting is not a sport—it's a spirit.

CHAPTER 1

THE DEATH SENTENCE

"If you're going through hell,
keep going."

Winston Churchill

FIGHT FACT

● ●

VICTORY IS ALWAYS POSSIBLE FOR THE PERSON WHO REFUSES TO STOP FIGHTING.

–Napoleon Hill

"GET READY TO SPEND the rest of your life in a wheelchair."

Nothing can ever prepare you for such life-changing news. I sat there stunned and frightened to death as the doctor rattled on about treatments, medication, and a very dismal diagnosis. It was permanent. It was incurable and terminal. And my quality of life would quickly start slipping away.

What was just as shocking to me as the diagnosis was how it was even possible. I was a pretty healthy person. I had always exercised regularly. I ate good foods. I didn't smoke. There wasn't any family history of multiple sclerosis (MS) that I could recall. I was only fifty-five years of age—a very active wife, mother, and grandmother. Sure, I wasn't going to be training for the Olympic games anytime soon, but I certainly wasn't old enough to be worrying about any major illnesses. Heck, I had the best years ahead of me, or so I thought. And yet here I was, in a cold and impersonal doctor's office, listening to some stranger in a white coat tell me that my life was basically over. And to add insult to injury, just days before I had been at the beach enjoying a vacation with my family. Talk about a slap in the face.

In June of 2004, I had taken my mother and her sister to Tybee Island in Georgia for a week. During the trip, I noticed that my neck was hurting constantly. I thought it was stress or maybe that I had thrown out my alignment during one of the many walks on the beach. Just one misstep is sometimes all it takes to aggravate a muscle. All I needed to do was relax and it would work itself out, which I was almost certain of.

The night after I returned home from vacation, I awoke with a tremendous pain in the back of my skull. It radiated down my entire left side, leaving me unable to move or even blink my eyes. The pain was so intense, it seemed as though it took an hour to force myself into a sitting position. When I realized this wasn't just some aggravated muscle, I woke up my husband, because I knew something was dreadfully wrong.

The ambulance arrived, and the EMTs had to take me out sitting straight up, since I couldn't move. At that time, we didn't know if I'd had an aneurysm or a stroke. What we did know was that I was in bad shape. I was brought to the hospital, given enough pain medication to take down a horse, and was released after several hours with a diagnosis of a probable pinched nerve. But I knew it was more than that, so I followed up with my primary care physician at Massachusetts General Hospital, who then referred me to the head of neurology for testing.

After a series of MRIs, a lumbar puncture, and other neurological tests, I went to see the neurologist for the test results. I truly didn't expect to hear anything bad as I sat across the desk from the doctor, anticipating some easily treatable diagnosis. Instead he said, "I have reviewed your tests, and you have multiple sclerosis. You need to prepare yourself for life in a wheelchair."

That was a defining moment in my life. My very survival had been threatened, and I had to choose between fight or flight. I could go home, get my affairs in order, and accept this sentence as though it were written in stone, slowly fading away until I was a shell of my true self, but that went against every fiber of my headstrong being.

> *I would do everything I could to hang on to a good quality of life and to search for answers.*

I didn't know much about MS, but I knew I didn't want to spend the rest of my life confined to a wheelchair. I was numb and overwhelmed with a million questions, but I knew I didn't want to die. I would do everything I could to hang on to a good quality of life and to search for answers.

Diagnosis be damned. The fight was on.

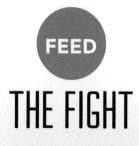

THE FIGHT

KNOWLEDGE TO SHARE WITH OTHERS

One study suggests that Patient Safety Incidents, which include misdiagnoses, "was the most common cause of a patient safety incident, with a rate of 155 per 1,000 hospitalized patients . . . and misdiagnosis rates in the ICU or Emergency Department have been studied, with rates ranging from 20% to 40%."
www.rightdiagnosis.com/intro/common.htm

Since very little is known about MS, here are three great websites for the latest updates and research:

**www.nationalmssociety.org/research/
research-news/index.aspx**

**www.msif.org/global-ms-research/
latest-ms-research-news/**

**www.sciencedaily.com/news/health_medicine/
multiple_sclerosis/**

CHAPTER 2

FIGHTING THE GOOD FIGHT

"Many people fail not so much because of their mistakes; they fail because they are afraid to try."

George Foreman III

FIGHT FACT

● ●

INTRODUCTION TO FIGHT LAW.

EVERY TIME I TOLD MY DAD that I was having a problem in college, work, or life in general, he always told me: "Just fight!" I did and I still do—I never give up—but I felt like that approach doesn't always work. I wanted more than two words and a smile. I wanted some substance! I mentioned that to him one day—that "just fight" seemed like polite encouragement rather than a roadmap for change. His response: "That's because you don't know how to fight." Ouch. What do you say to that?

Trying to save face, I said, "Of course I don't. I'm an academic, not a pugilist." Wrong answer.

Then he really let me have it. He said my attitude was why I never accomplished the things I thought I was fighting for, and if I was going to achieve anything of value in this world, I was going to have to fight for it—plain and simple. He explained that fighting is very simple, as long as I understand the principles of fighting and stick to them.

Sounded like good advice to me. So I asked a few more questions, hoping for the one secret—the answer to make it all click into place. Instead, he said I have to find my own answer. "The more you figure this out on your own, the more it will become a part of you."

And then, like a good coach, he gave me homework. "Find some video footage of the greatest fighters, and study what separates them from the fighters you have never heard of. You will quickly learn the principles of fighting, all of which apply in countless ways to health, wealth, and happiness." So I did.

After hours of studying ESPN Classic films and a lot of thought about what it really means to be a fighter, I discovered twelve lessons—life lessons, really—that when applied, separate the greats from the nameless.

THE MORE YOU FIGURE THIS OUT ON YOUR OWN, THE MORE IT WILL BECOME A PART OF YOU.

The greats aren't just found in the ring, either. Mary is a also true champion, fighting the Good Fight.

FIGHT LAW 1

THE GREATS NEVER GIVE UP.

GREAT FIGHTERS have a glaring will to win that seems to carry them through everything that should be a setback. They constantly employ different methods of imposing their will on their opponents, whether it is the face-off before the fight, standing up between rounds instead of sitting on the stool, standing over their opponent when they knock them down, screaming, or taking hard hits and hitting right back with no hesitation. Some even bounce up and down in the twelfth round when they should surely be ready to collapse from fatigue.

When I've asked great fighters why they do this, they always explain that it fills them with energy and renews their confidence. Just like Mary screams "YOU GO GIRL!", a battle cry—a show of resilience and will to live in the face of defeat—will often renew you with the confidence and energy to pull through your fight in the end.

CHAPTER 3

THE FIGHT OF MY LIFE

"In three words, I can sum up everything I've learned about life: It goes on . . . and I refuse to watch it go lying down."

●

Mary McAlary

FIGHT FACT

● ●

FIGHTERS KEEP ON FIGHTING THROUGH THE PAIN.

THE SIX WEEKS FOLLOWING the diagnosis were grueling. I was hospitalized for five days and put on an intravenous line of prednisone* to treat the inflammation that was contributing to the pain and lack of feeling in my body. The anti-inflammatory benefits of the prednisone were supposed to relieve my symptoms, but I had an allergic reaction to the medication—I very rarely took any kind of medicine. Within minutes of the medicine entering my bloodstream, I began to lose my breath and my speech softened to a mere whisper. Thankfully a friend was with me because I was unable to call for help. The doctors added Benadryl and Ativan at a very slow drip for the next five days, in order for my body to tolerate the medication. The numbness and pain did continue but eased somewhat. Still, for someone who considers herself to be a healthy person, this was a monumental shift and my body was thrown into overdrive.

Prednisone is used to treat conditions such as arthritis, blood disorders, breathing problems, severe allergies, skin diseases, cancer, eye problems, and immune system disorders. Prednisone belongs to a class of drugs known as corticosteroids.

When I was released, a nurse from the MS Society visited me at home to teach me how to inject myself with Betaseron*. It would make me very ill between injections with nausea and flu-like symptoms. I would have to take this every other day for the rest of my life. I hated the thought of feeling so sick every day, but surely the doctors knew what was best for me.

I developed large dark welts where the injections were given in my mid-stomach and thighs. After several weeks, there was nowhere to inject myself that was not dark, swollen, and sore. I was miserable. I was experiencing dry heaves and extreme fatigue. They were right—I constantly felt like I had the flu, and every time I would start to feel better, it was time for another shot. It quickly got to the point where I refused to give myself the shots and my husband would have to give them to me instead.

This was not how I wanted my family to see me.

This was not how I wanted my family to see me. My two younger children were teenagers then, and although they'd felt a little better after a private consultation with the doctor, seeing their mom sick and miserable was really tough on them. After all, their mother was now "disabled."

Some days, the only ray of sunshine I experienced was my daughter's puppy—a Westie named Marley. When I was lying there feeling hopeless, Marley would coax me into playing with her, taking her for walks, and most of all, she would make me smile. She had an uncanny sixth sense to know exactly where I was in pain, and she would put her

---

Betaseron is part of the Interferon Betas class and treats multiple sclerosis. Interferon betas are used to treat multiple sclerosis by helping the body fight viral infections.

head down at the very spot to warm it and soothe me. She was a little fur ball of blessings, but she could only do so much.

After several months of injections, I was lying on the couch one day and all of a sudden, I could almost hear my body pleading with me: *Stop taking the medication. It's just making you more ill.* Well that didn't make any sense. But the more I thought about it, the more I felt like I was having an internal conversation with my conscience.

"I'm sick. I need this medicine to stay healthy."

And just how well is that working for you?

"Good point."

I had to admit I wasn't feeling any better and the "quality of life" this medicine was supposed to give me was no real quality at all. I wasn't living; I was merely existing.

Something had to change. It had to change now. And you know what they say: If you want something done right, do it yourself.

I immediately stopped injecting the Betaseron and decided to seek out a new neurologist who would understand my concerns and support my decision, since my original doctor, whom I had started seeing after being referred to Brigham Hospital (since Mass. General does not treat MS) was very displeased when I told him I quit the medication.

That process took a lot longer than I expected. But my efforts paid off in more ways than I could have imagined. Not only did I begin to feel better, but I dove headfirst into seeking out every piece of information and research I could find about MS and treatment options. And I found a great doctor—a partner in this fight—who supported me every step of the way.

Finally, we were getting somewhere.

FIGHT LAW 2

GREAT FIGHTERS ALWAYS THROW THE FIRST PUNCH.

YOU CAN'T WIN unless you're in the fight, and you're not in the fight until you have thrown your first punch. This is often the hardest part, but once you throw it, your training, preparation, and the will to fight will do the rest of the work.

Mary's first punch was the risk of listening to her body and believing—against all odds, with MS being an incurable disease—that she could fight to get well.

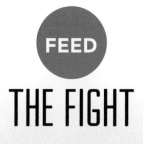

THE FIGHT

KNOWLEDGE TO SHARE WITH OTHERS

"Fighter's (as everyone should) must always know exactly what they are putting into their bodies. I am not saying what a person should or should not take, but I am saying that we should all know the consequences (positive or negative) of what we put into our bodies before we make the decision to do so."
—George Foreman III

Benadryl side effects
www.allergies.emedtv.com/benadryl/benadryl-side-effects.html

Ativan side effects
www.rxlist.com/ativan-drug.htm

Betaseron side effects
www.betaseron.com/safety/possible-side-effects

Prednisone side effects
www.drugs.com/sfx/prednisone-side-effects.html

CHAPTER 4

YOU'VE GOT TO FIGHT . . .
TO EDUCATE YOURSELF

"Our greatest
weakness lies in giving up.
The most certain way to succeed
is always to try just one
more time."

●

Thomas A. Edison

FIGHT FACT

• •

FIGHTERS ALWAYS HAVE A GAME PLAN, RESEARCHING TO DISCOVER THEIR OPPONENT'S WEAKNESSES.

I SAW FIVE DIFFERENT NEUROLOGISTS during the course of my search. Some didn't have the time, desire, or experience to answer the hundreds of questions I had in the beginning. To be fair, they weren't all trying to brush me off as some high-maintenance patient. In reality, very little is known about multiple sclerosis, which literally means "many scars" or "many lesions." When one has multiple sclerosis, the location of the lesions in the brain affects the parts of the body directly related to that location. In my case, it is very painful, attacking my nerve pain center.

The lack of knowledge about the disease made those early medication discussions even scarier. When I was first diagnosed, the doctors gave me my choice—yes, my choice—of five or six different medications, asking me which one I would prefer. *Well, how in the hell am I supposed to know which medication would be best? Aren't you the one with the degree?* It seemed backward to me. I was the patient; they were the doctors. It was very frightening to realize that my care and medical choices were completely up to me when I had no training and no in-depth knowledge about multiple sclerosis or pharmaceuticals. But that fear turned into liberation once I accepted that my health—my future—was up to me. And let's be honest, I had a lot more time on my hands to care about my well-being than they did anyway.

A doctor named Revere Philip Kinkel at Beth Israel Hospital in Boston, Massachusetts, would become one of my most trusted friends and supporters. He took the time to speak with me about multiple sclerosis and my options, and listened to my opinions and decisions about my choices. He was very supportive, telling me that as long as I did not develop any more lesions, he would stand by me. I'm happy to report he's still standing by me.

My hope is to encourage you to first strengthen your body with whole foods, healthy environments, and physical activity ...

Now I am not advocating that people suffering from diseases should stop taking their medication like I did. If you're battling an illness, you know just how overwhelming it is to be uncomfortable and to keep track of medications. While it is certainly a choice you may feel led to consider, my hope is to encourage you to first strengthen your body with whole foods, healthy environments, and physical activity, if possible, so that you are better able to fight disease while making important decisions about your health. As you get stronger physically, you will be better able to listen to your own body and find your own answers. I'm just here to remind you that you have options, and that you should have some expectations.

Remember, you're paying for care and treatment options. That means you should have some expectation of getting better or feeling better. Right? What's the sense in paying someone to help you slowly decline and still feel miserable the whole way down? I could do that by eating fast food three times a day, and it would be a lot cheaper.

If you feel like you're not getting the answers or the results you want, jump ship! Yes, it's scary. It's probably uncharted waters—thinking you have a say in your health care. But let's be honest ... you can't pay someone enough money to truly care about your well-being even more than you care about yourself.

You might never have realized that you can get a second or third or even a fifth opinion from a doctor. But you can. You may never have considered that there might be perfectly good natural substitutes for some medications. But there are. You may have been sick and miserable for so long that you've forgotten what having any shred of control over your life feels like. But there's hope. There's always hope. Some days, that's all I had.

While I was weaning myself off of the remaining medications, it seemed like it was hit or miss at times. Sometimes I did have to take new medications to cope with my body's reactions, and some produced very unpleasant side effects such as depression, mood changes, and fatigue.

The nerve pain was still severe, and I still had numbness and weakness. In order to alleviate the nerve pain, I was prescribed large doses (up to fourteen pills per day, at times) of a bipolar medication believed to be helpful in controlling neuropathy. Then I tried a drug called amitriptyline* that made me angry all the time, which is not my personality. I quickly decided that amitriptyline was not for me. This was followed by many other drugs in that same family, all of which had undesirable side effects. But when the pain got unbearable, I did agree to take them. I could only do—and stand—so much.

There were times I would find myself flat on my back on the floor, staring up at the ceiling, wondering how I fell without any warning. Sometimes when I walked, I would drag my feet, which would cause me to trip or be uneasy on my feet. There were other times when I was unable to take the short walk to my mailbox.

I developed restless leg syndrome, which would keep me awake all night long, unable to sleep, with spasms in my legs. In order to help me sleep, I was given sleeping pills. Then I developed spasms throughout my body and was prescribed another medication that made me feel even worse. Then I developed trigeminal neuralgia, a very painful condition in the chin area that feels like lightning is striking your face at the touch of the softest breeze or slightest mist. If I even tried to go outside, I'd have to cover that side of my face so that it felt no sensation from the weather. It was difficult and painful to shower, brush my teeth, eat, and sometimes even speak. So they gave me yet another medication. I was a mess.

Even though I felt I was moving in the right direction, I was steadily deteriorating. The medications caused depression and severe mood swings. I never knew from one day to the next what

---

Tricyclic antidepressants work by increasing levels of the mood chemicals serotonin and norepinephrine in the brain. Although amitriptyline is only licensed for use in depression, it is commonly prescribed "off-licence" to help ease certain types of nerve pain, and also to help prevent migraines.

I was going to be facing. As you can imagine, I was difficult to live with, and my family was also suffering right along with me. They couldn't fix me. They didn't always know how to help me—or even if they could help.

Finally, after seeing me change so drastically and decline so severely, and knowing that I was in no shape to fight anymore, my oldest daughter, Kristian, did her best to fight for me by giving me an ultimatum.

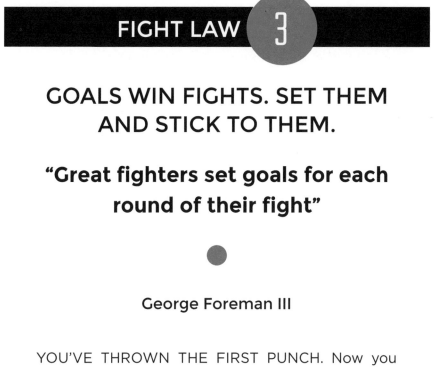

FIGHT LAW 3

GOALS WIN FIGHTS. SET THEM AND STICK TO THEM.

"Great fighters set goals for each round of their fight"

George Foreman III

YOU'VE THROWN THE FIRST PUNCH. Now you take time to study your challenge, to see what works and what doesn't. You look for opportunities you can exploit and pitfalls you must be cautious of for the rest of the fight.

In Mary's case, she had to educate herself about her opponent—the disease of MS—and learn new ways to do battle when old ways failed. In your case, you've most likely identified your opponent. Now you need to write down the game plan and test the waters.

In boxing, fighters only go for a knockout in the first round if they know that their capabilities and strength are far superior to that of their opponent, or if they are convinced they don't have what it takes to go twelve rounds. The first round is the most dreaded and often the most awkward, and 9 times out of 10, nothing major will occur in the first round. But fighters don't get discouraged. They take notes and amend their game plan as needed.

Remember that the first round is only a learning experience to prepare you for the rest of the fight. Plan your work and work your plan, making adjustments where needed.

THE FIGHT

KNOWLEDGE TO SHARE WITH OTHERS

So how can you get the most out of your doctors visit?

Prepare a list of questions or concerns ahead of time and also bring a list of current medications, known family conditions, and known allergies.

Ask questions if you don't understand or need clarification on specifics.

Write information down or record it on your phone. If you don't feel at ease, find another doctor for a second or third opinion. (Check to see what your options are with insurance. Also look online for reviews.)

CHAPTER 5

MARY'S FIGHT ANALOGY

"Always maintain your dignity; it will sweeten your adversity."

George Foreman III

FIGHT FACT

● ●

THIS OLE DOG HAS A FEW TRICKS UP HER SLEEVE.

IT IS ALL ABOUT THE BALANCE IN LIFE, which is never easy to attain. Just when everything seems to be going smoothly, another challenge presents itself. When times were tough for me, I used to tell my friends that this was how I felt:

> I am a dog off the leash and enjoying the freedom. I am walking down the road in complete euphoria when BANG, I get hit by a car. I'm hurt badly, but I decide to pick myself up, crawl to the side of the road, and wait until I am feeling well again. Great, I made it. . . .

> I cautiously set off down the road again, renewing my spirit. Yeah, I made it and I feel great! BOOM, I get hit by a bus. Now I am really hurt. I remember the past injuries and how hard it was for me to get up and get to the side of the road to heal. Can I do that again? Yes, I want to try again. So I painfully pick myself up and crawl to the side of the road to heal. It takes even longer this time because I am tired of all of this pain and disappointment, but I made it. I'm back on the road.

Now I figure this just can't happen again. Lightning is only supposed to strike once, not twice, so I begin again with a renewed spirit. I set out down that road, the sun shining on my face, a little sorer than before but determined to make it to the end of the road, and then CRASH, there's the Mack truck!

That is the moment when you know if you are a true fighter or not. The moment to decide whether to give in and die, or struggle through the pain, grasp onto LIFE, and survive because deep down inside you know you will win. I pick myself up again, crawl to the side of the road, aware that I may never fully heal. But this time it is different because I am no longer afraid to get hit; I know I will survive.

I am prancing down that road right now, head up high, with a bit of a limp, headed wherever it takes me.

There are passions in our lives that are a direct result of learning experiences. You can choose to ignore these passions or take action. I know that, through my passions, I have helped to save many lives. I pray that my passions change the lives of many of my brothers and sisters in this world. We all have a higher purpose that we need to fulfill. Mine is to help people. I know this because this makes my heart soar and my spirit feel fulfilled.

Whatever your passion is, find your path and follow it. Everybody fights. The question is, what do you fight for? My passion is to teach others how to fight through organic healthy, eating.

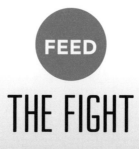

THE FIGHT

KNOWLEDGE TO SHARE
WITH OTHERS

One of the published side effects of aspartame is brain seizures in monkeys. Many humans personally report the same experiences. Always read the label of synthetic sweeteners before using them.
Our recommendation is pure stevia.

www.thehealthyhomeeconomist.com/aspartame-with-milk-may-trigger-brain-seizures/

CHAPTER 6

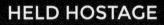

HELD HOSTAGE

"You have not lived today
until you have done something
for someone who can
never repay you."

●

John Bunyan

FIGHT FACT

• •

FIGHT FOR WHAT (OR WHO) YOU LOVE.

WHEN SOMEONE DEVELOPS A CHRONIC ILLNESS, it's normal for family or friends to hover around them for the first few weeks or months, trying to help. Time goes on and their attention and patience wane. Yes, being so sick is physically and emotionally draining. But it can be just as draining to be a constant caregiver. After a while, people go on with their lives.

It was the same for my family. They were going out, seeing people, and enjoying life. I felt like a shut-in, completely isolated from the world around me, and terribly sad. Even when they were around, I was unable to interact with them or play with my grandchildren the way I used to. I would just sit on my couch and my daughter would hand the baby to me for short periods of time. My other grandchildren would just sit and stare at me, wondering what happened to their fun-loving and energetic Grammy.

My condition and the medications that I was still taking had started to take a toll on my appetite. Eating had become difficult because I was almost always nauseous from the medication. Most of the time, I just didn't eat, although when I did, I ate what I believed to be a balanced, healthy diet.

Kristian saw what was happening, and she'd had enough. She had discovered a passion for healthy eating in high school after having brain seizures that were linked to the aspartame in diet sodas. She stopped drinking diet sodas and the seizures stopped. To this day, she reads every label to make sure that it does not contain aspartame (or any of its other many names), and it is banned in her home and in mine.

When she gained weight after giving birth to her second child, she began running, exercising, and working on her diet and is now one of the fittest people I know. Several years later, when the school told her that it was a possibility that her daughter had a learning disability and might need medication, Kristian decided to seek a holistic approach to avoid any medications. She believed that there was a better "alternative" and began feeding her healthier foods. Her daughter never went on medication and is doing great in school.

That passion for food awareness led Kristian to enroll in the Institute for Integrative Nutrition (IIN) in 2006. She began advising me to eat foods that I had never really paid attention to before, such as quinoa, buckwheat, flax oil, kale, and other whole foods (those that have not been altered in any way from their natural state). Of course, she'd been telling me about these foods for a while. I just hadn't listened.

Kristian knew that the medicine wasn't helping me get well, but if I gave healthy eating an honest chance, it would change my life. She would tell me that miracles could happen just by changing my diet, and I would roll my eyes at her. After all, I grew up in a farming area, and as a child, I had spent many hours helping out on neighbors' farms.

Still, when I was hesitant to listen or make any changes to my diet, she demanded that I apply for the 2007 classes at Institute for Integrative Nutrition (IIN) so that I could see firsthand what she had been trying to tell me for the past year. And to make sure her point stuck, she actually threatened to disown me if I did not apply to the school. Talk about a low blow. I had grandkids to spoil! I couldn't be disowned. You've heard the saying that all is fair in love and war, right? Well, that's a lie.

At that time, I carried a cane in case I needed support to walk. I sure as heck didn't believe that I would be capable of going to New York in the condition I was in or be able to attend sixteen hours of classes per weekend for ten months. But I didn't want to be disowned, either. I love my grandkids too much.

So I applied to IIN under threat of mental anguish, and I purposely did it very late—that way I could keep my promise to my daughter and I wouldn't have to worry about getting in. (Kristian never said I had to apply early or on time.) I was number eighty-eight on a waiting list of one hundred people, so I relaxed. I did, however, promise myself, my daughter, and God that if, by chance and against all odds, I did get accepted, I would go because I knew that a higher power had made that decision for me—one that I couldn't ignore.

On the final day to be accepted to the program, I was eating dinner, not sure whether I was disappointed because I didn't get the call or happy that I didn't get the call. That's when the phone rang.

I was accepted to the program! I took it as a sign of better things to come. Little did I know at that time the remarkable change that one decision would have on my life.

FIGHT LAW 4

PAIN IS THE MIDDLE NAME OF A GREAT FIGHTER'S GAME.

YOU ONLY HAVE A CHANCE of winning the fight if you're in it. But you must understand that, in a fight, there will be damage. In boxing, that comes in the form of bruises, cuts, body aches, broken bones, swollen eyes and face, illegal headbutts and punches, and of course, the dreaded knockdown.

In life, the fight may be overcoming situations that seem impossible or in dealing with pain so severe that it challenges your will to move forward. You must stay determined to get back up and continue your journey.

YOU MUST STAY DETERMINED TO GET BACK UP AND CONTINUE YOUR JOURNEY.

All of this is okay, as it comes with the territory. The only way this can be negative is if you quit because of a setback. If you have not experienced any of the damage—physically or mentally—then you'd better reevaluate what you are doing because odds are that you are not in the fight.

You also have to remember that you never fight alone. Those who are observing you during your fight are also looking closely to see how you handle setbacks, and it is important that those who will be instrumental in your success see that nothing breaks your will or weakens your resolve to continue the fight. How you fight will inspire others.

Likewise, your opponents will be watching like hawks to see one inch of weakness in your countenance when you experience setbacks, so that they can exploit these opportunities. Make sure that the only thing they perceive is a renewed sense of urgency and determination to win; it will surely deter theirs.

Mary encountered this struggle in her own fight. So many times, people doubted her choices and paths to wellness, but she didn't allow anything or anyone to break her resolve. She says, "I will do everything I can to 'live' my life."

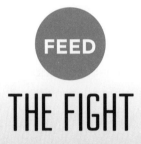

THE FIGHT

KNOWLEDGE TO SHARE WITH OTHERS

Drink your way to health.

Our bodies are made of 55 to 80 percent water, so it's important that we drink enough to stay hydrated. We used to hear that we needed 8 glasses of water a day, and while that's a great start, depending on your weight, you may need more. A good rule of thumb is to divide your weight in half and then drink that many ounces per day.

CHAPTER 7

NEW YORK CITY BY FORCE

**"Courage is being scared
to death—and saddling
up anyway."**

John Wayne

FIGHT FACT

● ●

IT ISN'T ABOUT HOW MANY TIMES YOU GET KNOCKED DOWN, BUT HOW MANY TIMES YOU GET BACK UP.

IN EARLY OCTOBER 2007, on a Friday, I got into my car and headed to my daughter's house. The following day, I would be starting my first day of school. On Saturday morning, the roles were totally reversed, and just as I had done so many years ago, my daughter woke me up before dawn, telling me to get ready. She and my grandchildren had packed me a lunch of quinoa wrapped in collard greens and sent me off to school.

Like many students on the first day of school, I was frightened to death! My stomach was a massive knot, and I could not believe that just weeks before my fifty-ninth birthday, I was headed to Manhattan. What was I thinking?

I had not been in New York City for years, and frankly I was a bit apprehensive about being in the city by myself, especially after 9/11. But there I was, my cane sitting next to me on the front seat of the car.

The sun had begun to rise just as I crossed onto the Henry Hudson Parkway. For some reason, when I saw the skyline of Manhattan lit up by the morning sun, I got an incredible feeling of elation! I blasted my radio, opened my sunroof, and yelled, "You go, girl!" into the wind. There are no words to convey the profound confidence, hope, and joy that I felt at that particular moment. I just knew I was finally doing something healthy for myself.

The classes at the Institute for Integrative Nutrition were like going to a full day of the *Oprah* show. From 8 a.m. to 4 p.m., there was music, a great atmosphere, classes, and an instant camaraderie with the other students in that large arena at the Lincoln Center. Our guest lecturers—John Doulliard, Dr. Oz, Andrew Weil, Mark Hyman, Deepak Chopra, and many others—were some of the top experts in the nutrition field. I was so excited to be there! And as pumped up as I now was about the classes, my husband was a bit more skeptical.

To be honest, I think that my husband, Fred, thought I was crazy when I decided to go to IIN. He thought the rigorous schedule on those weekends would not be good for me. I was, after all, disabled and not doing really well. But he also knew me well enough to know that once I set my mind to something, it is next to impossible to change it, so he just accepted it.

When I started school that first weekend, I was still unsteady on my feet, very tired, and was barely managing the nerve pain levels. I was on eighteen medications at that time, including Ambien to help me sleep. Sunday morning, after my very first day of classes, I awoke around 12:30 a.m., got out of bed, and headed to the bathroom. It was dark and I was a bit dazed from the sleep-aid. Suddenly I misstepped, crashed down two flights of stairs, and stopped rolling just outside of my daughter's bedroom door. I had landed on my left wrist and shattered it. On top of that, I was bruised and bleeding and looked like I had been hit by a truck.

My daughter called the ambulance, and I was taken to the local hospital. I would need emergency surgery as soon as possible. Still, with all the pain and confusion of the night, I could not believe that I had to miss school the next day after all I'd gone through to get this far! Determined to recover as quickly as possible, I had the surgery and now have a titanium wrist to forever remind me of my first day at school. That Sunday was my only absence throughout the program.

While it certainly wasn't convenient or pleasant, that accident changed my health in a very positive way. My daughter held me captive at her house for several weeks after the surgery, since I could not be moved back to mine. Now she had me right where she wanted me and was able to basically force me to eat healthy, whole foods. The horror!

About a week after my wrist surgery (and a week of eating whole foods), I had just finished lunch when I realized that I felt incredibly better from the inside out. It was almost as if someone had given me a shot of good health and energy—a thousand times better than the shots I had never grown accustomed to at the beginning of my diagnosis. Even though I was in a great deal of pain, I felt a transformation beginning within. It was a revelation, to say the least.

To be honest, the healthy foods weren't bad tasting or expensive, as I'd assumed. In fact, they were refreshing and delicious. Realizing the impact of the foods on my well-being, healing, and mood, I began to experiment with different types of nutritional eating. The more I learned about nutrition, the more I craved healthier foods.

I also worked very hard to learn to manage my stress levels, spending many hours listening to meditation tapes geared toward relaxation and healing. I found this to be a very important part of my healing process, because with all the big and sudden changes I had experienced in the last few years—and throughout my life—I certainly had a lot of stress!

It's pretty common knowledge these days that stress causes many illnesses and can certainly delay the healing process. When you're stressed out, your adrenal system is attacked and leaves you more vulnerable to disease by lowering your immune responses. It also affects your mood, which spills over to your work, your family, your friends, and your self-image. We live in a world of constant stress—and it can't always be avoided. But we need to learn to manage it so that it does not harm us. For me, rest and relaxation did wonders.

Another very important aspect of my recovery was increasing my intake of water. It's such a simple change to your daily life, but I cannot stress enough how important it is to stay hydrated. Our bodies consist of 55 to 80 percent water. We can live for weeks without food, but only days without water. It's pretty darn important.

I cannot stress enough how important it is to stay hydrated. Our bodies consist of 55 to 80 percent water.

I was never a water drinker. I never craved it; I never even thought about it. I got my "water" intake for the day through other drinks and foods. But as I began to drink more water, I began to feel better. I could feel the changes within me, and I was eager to see what the next nine months of classes and healthy eating would accomplish. I was keeping my promise, even if it healed me.

FIGHT LAW 5

GREAT FIGHTERS LISTEN TO THEIR CORNER.

IF YOU ARE PRIVILEGED enough to have a good mentor to confide in, make sure you listen to them in the heat of the battle. Find a good mentor that you can trust and listen to them. For Mary, that person was her daughter, Kristian, who led the way for her and still does to this day. The support of her husband and children has also been critical to her ability to fight.

In the fight, if you are passionate, your emotions will most likely cloud your judgment from time to time. This is good! It means that you are serious about winning. But you must remember that this is when you need to listen to the objective voice of your mentor, who will be your voice of reason when you are too consumed with passion to think clearly. We all have an inner voice, but some of us don't listen to it or trust it. Most of the time, it is telling you the same things your mentors will.

And remember, only take advice from other great fighters. You and you alone determine which voices you allow to speak into your life. How do you know they are great fighters? Look at their record of success.

CHAPTER 8

NEVER FORGET
YOUR FIGHT

"Those who know, do.
Those that understand, teach."

Aristotle

FIGHT FACT

● ●

EVERY FIGHTER
NEEDS A TRAINER.

WHEN YOU ARE FINISHING up classes at IIN, they encourage you to begin counseling others in holistic health matters. I began coaching people in the spring of 2008. I was excited to reinvent myself and share my knowledge with others. Since then, I've helped hundreds of people make the steps toward healthy eating and an active lifestyle.

I was also determined to reach out to the MS community and continue my education and research. When I was first diagnosed with multiple sclerosis, I was told not to tell anyone because I could lose my job and people would treat me differently. Well, I've never been the kind of person to keep things from people—I wear my heart on my sleeve. I also feel that the more people who know about multiple sclerosis, the more funding may become available to fight this insidious disease. So I chose to speak out. When I began sharing about my disease, I was shocked to find out how many people either had it as well or knew someone who did. That only convinced me more that my life's purpose was to mentor others and help to bring awareness to the benefits of healthy living.

Through one-on-one mentoring, group coaching events, and radio and television interviews, I've been able to share my knowledge and make a positive impact on people's lives. I also really enjoy my work with the Esperanza Academy girls each year, teaching them about healthy eating. You can never be too young to learn how to eat right!

My goal when coaching people is to teach them to "listen" to their bodies and to eat healthy foods. I also encourage them to examine their "primary food" sources (such as healthy relationships and a balanced life) to make sure that every area is balanced. If you think about it, so many people eat (and make poor food choices) because of boredom and stress. But if those areas of their lives that make them unhappy were whole, that need to binge or fill an emptiness wouldn't exist.

I work with people who have conditions such as MS, cancer, Parkinson's disease, lupus, and autoimmune diseases. I also work with people who just want to feel better, lose weight, and be healthy. No matter the client's goal—or age—it is so gratifying to see lives changed by making good decisions.

One of my clients, Molly, was just sixteen years old when I met her. She had just been diagnosed with multiple sclerosis, and it was affecting her eyesight. Molly was a great tennis player on the high school tennis team, and as you can imagine, her damaged eyesight affected her performance, making it impossible for her to continue to play for her team. She's such a vibrant young woman, and I wanted her to experience the best life has to offer. So I started by teaching her about organic foods.

With any program, in order for it to be sustainable, it's best to start it slowly so it isn't overwhelming. The trick with Molly was to begin to introduce healthy alternatives of the foods that she was already eating to show her that organic foods did taste good—most even tasted better than the unhealthy foods she was eating.

We agreed on a six-month program, changing the foods that she ate and doing some cooking together. Her sister, Michelle, joined us and provided Molly with great support throughout the program. The support of your family during these changes is a key to success. It only takes one person to sabotage a goal. Likewise, it only takes one person to stand beside you to provide support along the way.

It only takes one person to stand beside you to provide support along the way.

After those six months, Molly had improved and was able to rejoin the tennis team. For her senior project a few years later, she did an presentation about the harmful effects of aspartame, and I was very privileged to be her professional advisor throughout the project. I watched as she presented her paper to her class, feeling like a proud mother. She did an incredible job. So incredible, in fact, that she was asked to present the project to the school committee in her town to change the cafeteria programs of the schools in the district.

Molly is currently attending the University of New Hampshire, where she is majoring in neuroscience. She completed an internship this summer at the multiple sclerosis camp in Long Island, New York, working with pediatric multiple sclerosis patients. I know that one day she will help many others overcome neurological diseases such as MS, and she will forever be a believer in healthy eating because she witnessed the healing powers firsthand.

Another success story began while I was visiting my brother in Florida. His neighbor's daughter-in-law had been diagnosed with multiple sclerosis and was in a wheelchair. She has a little girl and a husband who need her and desperately wanted her to be well, so I agreed to see her that day and to continue to counsel her by telephone. After six months, she was out of the wheelchair and feeling better. The next time I visited my brother, she walked over to the house to hug me. Her husband had his wife back and their daughter was happy to have her mother back.

Everyone is different, every body is different, and it is up to us to determine what makes us the healthiest.

Everyone is different, every body is different, and it is up to us to determine what makes us the healthiest. Part of my job as a holistic health coach is to guide my clients through the process of finding out what's best for their unique bodies and give them the support they need to make the changes that will ensure they have optimal health.

As I said, this process does not happen overnight. I work with clients for six-month periods in order for them to begin to feel the changes in their bodies. I'm also able to give them the continued knowledge and support they need to try different approaches, and also to feel confident to continue to discover what is best for them.

Remember, it is never too late to change, re-create, and pursue new adventures. Your journey to wellness is waiting for you.

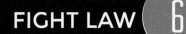

FIGHT LAW 6

GREATS NEVER TAKE
A ROUND OFF.

A FIGHT IS TWELVE ROUNDS, but the first and third rounds are just as important as the ninth and eleventh. A round off is a round lost.

In life or in business, if you take a day off, you can be sure you are taking a loss. You can bet your bottom dollar that when you take time off, not only are there others looking to take your spot, your opposition is gaining ground. And just like in a fight, they take it in pieces, like points.

Yes, life happens. There are always unforeseen events that will blindside you. But the key is to bounce back quickly. You can take a round off and still win, as long as you fight with the knowledge that you have given away points that can never be regained. That means you need to work even harder to get ahead.

Thankfully, each and every day is another opportunity to gain the necessary skills to continue your fight. Think of every day as a gift and a learning experience.

CHAPTER 9

●

THE POWER OF
ORGANIC EATING

"Let food be thy medicine and medicine be thy food."

Hippocrates

FIGHT FACT

• •

FIGHTERS FIGHT TO REACH A GOAL AND THEN WORK TO MAINTAIN IT.

NO ONE IS PERFECT. We all falter but the key is to strive to bounce back and try again. Most diets do not work because they are too restrictive. Just as soon as you're told you can't have something, that's exactly when you want it. You'll never want a piece of cake more in your life than the split-second after you've been told you can't have a slice because it will ruin your diet.

During my program, when I'm teaching people how to eat better, I add healthy foods to their diet. In time, their cravings for sugar and processed foods, which are so harmful, are eliminated. As they begin to get more energy and feel healthier, they seldom go back to wanting processed foods and are able to feel the difference in their bodies if they do eat them. Plus, if it's their idea and not mine that they don't really need to eat an entire carton of ice cream, it's much more likely to stick.

That's not to say that we all don't cheat now and then. We may choose to eat something we know may not be the most healthful —but that's part of life. If you had to avoid some of your favorite foods for the rest of your life in order to succeed, you'd never stick with a healthier food plan. And I couldn't blame you. Healthy eating isn't meant to be a punishment. It's really a blessing. And if you eat good foods most of the time, a less healthy choice every now and then is perfectly fine. Enjoy it!

This is where the 80/20 rule comes in: If you can eat well 80 percent of the time, the 20 percent spent eating foods that aren't as optimal is really okay. This gives everyone the license not to have to be perfect—the license to be human—and therefore, they are much less likely to give up on embracing a healthier diet and lifestyle.

There's also great power in finding balance in all areas of life. If you are generally happy and eat the healthiest foods possible at least 80 percent of the time, your chances of good health are great. If you are unhappy but eating well, you are still not balanced and could still be at risk for stress-related illnesses. If you are happy in your life but don't eat well, your chances for good health are also at risk. Finding your unique balance is key to good health.

In America, we are an instant gratification society. We get a headache, so we pop a pill; we get a stomachache, so we reach for the Tums. When we get sick, the first thing we think about is which pill is going to make us better—not what we can eat to make our bodies better. We've forgotten that food is medicine!

By the time most people are senior citizens, they are taking many medications. So many, in fact, that we have plastic pill containers to help us arrange our pills for thirty days at a time! All of these medications have side effects, and some of the side effects require even more medication, until before long, like myself, you're taking eighteen pills per day and still not feeling well. That's a ridiculous amount of pills, and it's expensive, no matter what healthcare plan you have. This isn't normal even though our society and pharmaceutical companies would like for us to think it is. Thankfully, it doesn't have to be this way.

Hear me out: It is not my goal to eliminate medications that are critical to one's recovery or to life itself, but it is my goal to eliminate medications that are unnecessary and have harmful side effects, especially when they can be replaced by natural food and an active lifestyle.

On the next page, I've listed some tips to help you reclaim and maintain a healthy lifestyle.

FIGHT LAW 7

IN FIGHTING, YOUR BEST DEFENSE IS YOUR OFFENSE.

Always maintain a proactive mindset. You will never win a fight by constantly defending yourself. Stay positive.

A good offense will score points, confuse and discourage your opposition, and keep them in defensive mode, which reduces your need to defend, and prevents them from scoring. Don't be afraid to try new approaches. You might just come up with a sucker punch!

The best defense in the world cannot score points. You can only score with offense. A good offense will always make your opposition think twice about getting up, going another round, or stepping into the ring at all. As your strength grows, your opponent's lessens. Don't take "no" for an answer. Be proactive.

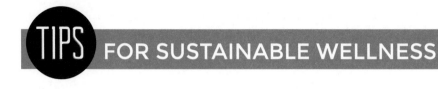

TIPS FOR SUSTAINABLE WELLNESS

1 Use alternatives to processed sugars, such as agave nectar, brown rice syrup, maple syrup, blackstrap molasses, and others.

2 Only use all-natural, organic sweeteners like pure stevia.

3 Beware of antibacterial soaps, especially those containing triclosan.

4 If you are taking medications, please read the side effects of the drugs. Many times, you can confuse these side effects with symptoms you may be experiencing.

5 Read labels. If you don't know what the ingredients are, don't eat it! Try to choose items that have five ingredients or less and are ones that you can identify.

6 Ask questions and don't stop until you are satisfied with the answers.

7 Think brown—brown rice, whole grains, products with unbleached flour and sugars, whole foods (those that haven't been altered from their natural state). Avoid white bread, white rice, and sugary cereals.

8 Try to find products with more fiber than sugar. This is a challenging scavenger hunt, but worth it.

9 Seek help and support to make the right choices for your body.

10 Have allergy testing to see what foods do not agree with you and should not be in your diet.

11 Don't be afraid to try new and different ways of eating. Try gluten-free, raw, or vegetarian diets, just to name a few, to see what's right for you.

12 Drink lots of water. The general rule is to divide your weight in half and aim to drink that many ounces each day.

13 Use household products without chemicals and those that are eco-friendly. Chemicals have an effect on your body whether ingested, inhaled, or absorbed through the skin.

14 Your skin is your largest organ. Feed it with healthy organic lotions, body products, and hair products.

15 Eat locally whenever possible.

16 Eat organic foods as much as possible. Learn which foods are the worst offenders (which contain the most pesticides) and spend the extra money, if necessary, on the organic types. It's cheaper in the long run than disease.

17 Learn how to clean your food before eating it. Wash your fruits and veggies well.

18 Partner with a few friends and encourage each other to eat healthier. Friends are a great support system.

19 Eat out less often. It is difficult to control what you are eating if you are not the chef. If you do eat out, seek out restaurants that serve healthy alternatives.

20 Remember, no one is perfect! Try to eat well 80 percent of the time and enjoy a cheat now and then. It is the quickest way to get back on track.

21 Listen to your body. It will let you know when it's happy and running well. A healthy body is in balance.

22 Eliminate stress. Stress causes illness! Ask yourself if this is worth getting sick about. If stress is unavoidable, try relaxation techniques or talk to someone to help you get through tough times.

23 Take care of your body so that it can take care of you. Feed it the best fuel and maintain it well with exercise, laughter, and rest.

24 Forgive. Harboring ill feelings does you more harm and gives that person power. You may feel they don't deserve to receive forgiveness, but you deserve to have freedom from the bitterness. Reclaim your heart.

25 Love yourself and be well.

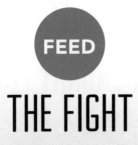

THE FIGHT

KNOWLEDGE TO SHARE WITH OTHERS

What do you need to know about triclosan?

It is believed that triclosan causes muscle weakness and breaks down the immune system. It is a possible link to neurological diseases. Below are three sites to visit to learn more.

www.examiner.com

www.wellnessdentalcare.com

www.abcnews.go.com

PRIMARY FOOD AND SECONDARY FOOD

As I mentioned earlier, healthy living is more than just food. There are primary and secondary sources that affect our bodies, minds, and relationships. According to the Institute for Integrative Nutrition (IIN):

> Primary food is more than what is on your plate. Healthy relationships, regular physical activity, a fulfilling career, and a spiritual practice can fill your soul and satisfy your hunger for life. When your primary food is balanced and satiating, your life feeds you, making what you eat secondary. . . .

> When we use secondary food as a way to alleviate or suppress our hunger for primary food, the body and mind suffer. Weight gain is just one of the consequences. Diet-related disorders such as heart disease, cancer, obesity, high blood pressure and diabetes are national epidemics, and one of the main reasons is because we are stuffing ourselves with secondary foods when we are really starving for primary food.*

---

*www.integrativenutrition.com/glossary/primary-food

My Personal Interpretation of Primary Food:

by Mary McAlary

- Primary food is the people in your life who support and love you through thick and thin.
- It is the feeling you get when you are in great shape physically and your body feels like a finely tuned engine.
- It is the peace you feel looking out over the ocean and hearing its waves washing your mind and healing your soul.
- It is the feeling of satisfaction you get when you know that you have done the best job you can possibly do and that you are appreciated.

Hold on to these good things and nurture them, while letting go of the unwelcomed stresses and unhealthy habits.

- Primary food is when you are surrounded by your children and grandchildren and know that they are all happy and healthy.
- Primary food is the look in your parents' and grandparents' eyes when they see you.
- It is looking into your spouse's eyes and seeing the love in them.
- It is that feeling that all is right in your world.
- It is unconditional love.
- If you can hold on to these good things and nurture them, while letting go of the unwelcomed stresses and unhealthy habits, you're well on your way to greater health.

CHAPTER 10

LEARN TO LOVE LEMONADE!

"Pattern recognition converts coincidence into meaning. Perpetual vigilance amidst experience begets genius. For it is in these moments that we discover our purpose."

●

George Foreman III

FIGHT FACT

● ●

FIGHTERS LEARN FROM EVERY SITUATION AND OUTCOME.

WHEN I FIRST SEE a client, I tell them that the first step to being well is to believe that you can be well. That commitment will bring you great strength.

I often use the analogy that our bodies are like our automobiles. If you put bad fuel in your automobile and don't maintain it, it breaks down and does not run its best. But our bodies, unlike our automobiles, cannot be traded in. We can certainly buy new parts with modern medicine—new knees, hips, artificial hearts, titanium wrists, and more. But obtaining these parts is a very painful process and also very expensive. Our bodies need to run on the best foods possible to experience tiptop performance. We require constant maintenance like exercise, rest, and occasional tune-ups. The better grade of food we eat, the better performance we achieve. It's ironic that the answer is right under our noses—it's our mouths.

I also believe that when you begin to make the right choices, you'll start to recognize patterns and symbols around you that can act as encouragement. When I was in tough shape, I was constantly noticing butterflies around me. Everywhere I went, they would land on me or fly around me, making themselves so visible. I looked up the symbolism of the butterfly and learned that it represents transformation. It was my time to transform my health and life. Now I use a butterfly as my logo for that reason.

I am also a very spiritual person. I was raised Catholic and attended first through eighth grade at St Joseph's School in Haverhill, Massachusetts. The nuns did their best to make the church my calling, and it nearly worked until I reached the eighth grade and had a crush on one of the boys. Though there was to be no nunhood for me, I have always had a deep faith in God. I believe my faith was a huge component of my recovery.

Treat others as you would like others to treat you, and always do your best to help others.

I believe that it is our responsibility to live by the Golden Rule: "Treat others as you would like others to treat you," and to always do your best to help others. My parents used to tell me that I always brought home stray dogs, cats, and people. I recognize that I have a need to help others. It is an important part of my makeup and makes me feel whole.

The volunteer work that I continue to do helps me to give back to my community. I was honored to be asked to sit on the Board of Delamano, Inc. and was elected president in 2007. I am very proud of the work I do fighting against domestic violence. It has become an epidemic in this country and around the world. My deepest passion is for the well-being of the children of these families and the innocent victims who deserve to live happy, peaceful lives. If people can live in peace, the world will be a healthier and happier place to live.

I am also continually amazed at how one gesture of kindness can go such a long way and circle back to where it came from.

Once I had committed to the classes at IIN, I decided to contact others from my area who were also enrolled. I sent an e-mail out after the first session to connect with people who were within fifteen miles of my home. My idea was to host meetings at my home where everyone could bring a healthy dish, share our thoughts about what we had learned, and support each other throughout the coming year at IIN.

The first meeting was right after our first weekend of class—the same weekend I broke my wrist. The doorbell rang and my first classmate had arrived. He was a twenty-something young man with a great smile. I didn't notice immediately that he had a disability too.

He asked me about the brace on my wrist, and I told him my story about falling down the stairs. At that point, he showed me his arm and told me that when he was three years old, he was on a lawn mower with his father.

I said, "And you fell off that lawnmower, didn't you?"

I will never forget the look of surprise on his face.

Then I asked, "Do you have an aunt named Carol?"

He did.

As it turned out, I had met Matt twenty years earlier.

I used to go to the gym with his aunt Carol every day, and she had shared his story with me after the accident. Matt ended up spending months in Massachusetts General Hospital Pediatric Rehabilitation. I felt so bad for him that, one day, I went to the hospital, brought him a teddy bear, and spent some time playing with him.

Matt remembered that bear. How amazing is that? What's even more amazing is that the same little boy would show up at my door more than twenty years later as a fellow student.

We commuted together throughout the entire experience, and he remains a special and inspirational person in my life. This is just one more example of how an act of kindness always comes back to you.

Though life has handed me many lemons throughout my years, I believe that when you experience difficult times, the best thing to do is to turn them into positive experiences. I am a fantastic lemonade maker!

FIGHT LAW 8

WHEN THE COMPETITION IS HURT OR HAS BEEN KNOCKED DOWN, GREAT FIGHTERS DO NOT GIVE THEM THE CHANCE TO RECOVER.

WHEN YOUR COMPETITION FALTERS, seize the moment and do everything you can to take them out of the fight or to make them quit. Never sacrifice your position of having the upper hand in the process.

This is truly a challenge regarding your health, because if you are feeling great, you may have a tendency to slip back into bad habits. At IIN, this is called sabotage.

Take notes! You can gain valuable wisdom about other competitors, and the events of their demise, which will supplement your knowledge and skills. Share your knowledge with others and remember to take the time to just listen as well.

TO BE HEALTHY

BELIEVE The first step to getting well is to believe that you can.

TRUST Trust your body to know what is best for you.

LISTEN Learn to listen to your body. It will tell you when something is wrong.

EXPLORE There are many dietary theories. Find out which ones may be right for you.

EXPERIMENT Don't be afraid to try new foods and new ways of eating.

LOVE We not only grow from food, we grow from relationships and caring. Falling in love feels wonderful.

PERSIST Never give up.

ENJOY Each day we are given is a gift. Live it to the best of your ability.

JOY Try each day to appreciate the joy in your life.

SING Sing a happy song every day, no matter how difficult that day may be. The song will begin to heal you.

MOVE	Try each day to move somehow. My dad would dance with me in his wheelchair—one of my fondest memories.
HUG	Share such a powerful way to say you care.
SMILE	Share a smile every day with someone. Smiles will return to you tenfold.
CRY	Never be afraid to cry. It is your body's way of releasing pain or experiencing great joy.
LAUGH	Release those endorphins!
PLAY	Let the child inside you come out.
BE UNCOMFORTABLE	Do something totally out of your comfort zone. When you do, you will gain confidence.
GIVE	Volunteer to help others. It is one of the most rewarding experiences you will ever have.
REST	We all need to recharge our internal batteries.
FIGHT	Fight for life, love, health, and happiness.

CHAPTER 11

FAITH: THE POWER OF INTENTION

"Great Champions have Great Faith.
Because to be a Champion,
you have to believe in yourself
when no one else will."

●

Sugar Ray Robinson

FIGHT FACT

• •

FIGHTERS THINK TO WIN.

I BELIEVE IN THE POWER of intention and feel that if you put your intentions out to the universe and make them known, sooner or later, those intentions somehow happen. I want to share a story with you about an intention I sent out to the universe.

I used to spend five or six weeks at a lovely beach in Kennebunkport, Maine, with my family. I met a wonderful woman who also visited every summer. She lived in California and had been coming to Maine every summer since she was a child. Her family owned a house in Kennebunk and when she didn't stay there, she stayed with her in-laws just a few doors down from the beach house that we leased.

We were going through many of the same struggles and spent hours walking the beach, talking and sharing. We buried parents, went through divorce, raised children, and both remarried. We kept in touch throughout the year and looked forward to seeing each other every summer. After my divorce, I continued to visit her each summer when she was in Maine.

Five years ago, she was diagnosed with breast cancer, which had also taken her mother years earlier. She decided to have a radical mastectomy. She underwent chemotherapy and radiation that made her very ill. It was a very difficult process, and at times, we were unsure if she would live.

For the first time since she was a child, she was unable to travel to Goose Rocks Beach and that was devastating for us both. It was so important for us to walk that beach each summer and share our triumphs and hardships.

That summer in her absence, I drove to Maine one morning. It was a cool day and no one else was on the beach. I walked the beach and began to cry for my friend. I decided to send a message. I picked up a broken shell with a sharp edge and wrote large letters into the sand: "Susan will get well and she will walk this beach again." I stayed until the water washed my message out to sea, into infinity and the powers beyond.

When I told Susan what I had done, we both cried and promised that the following summer she would be there. I am happy to say that Susan is healthy today, and we are back visiting and walking that beach each and every year.

As positive as intention can be, negativity can be equally as powerful and damaging. Two years after my diagnosis, I received an invitation from the MS Society to attend a golf outing for MS patients. I thought it would be a positive experience to meet other people with MS and be able to get some exercise while learning to golf.

I arrived early that day and found a tent set up with snacks and cold drinks. Several volunteers were setting up tees to hit, and I was given a club and some balls and began practicing. It was good to be outside and to learn something new.

People began arriving, some walking, and some in wheelchairs. They had special golf carts for those in wheelchairs, and it was wonderful to see how much they enjoyed the freedom to golf with those carts.

After the golfing was over, everyone sat under the tent enjoying a cold drink and conversation. One of the women turned to me and asked me how long ago I had been diagnosed. I told her that it had been two years. Then, instead of being positive, they all began to tell me that I should enjoy the time I had left, since they all were in wheelchairs five years after they found out they had MS. One said, "It was as if someone flipped a switch at that five-year mark and I went into this chair." At least six of them agreed, and I was just devastated. They may have meant well and were just trying to prepare me, but to me, it was a harsh sentence.

I got back to my car and burst into tears. Though I desperately wanted to be well and made every step I could toward a healthy life, what they said that day remained in my mind for the next three years. I was scared to death to reach my five-year mark and the possibility that I would wake up one day and need a wheelchair. I hoped that I had made the right decision when I stopped the medication. Only time would tell.

It has been over ten years since my diagnosis, and there's no wheelchair in sight. I don't mean to infer that life in a wheelchair is a death sentence or the worst of circumstances. I have the utmost respect for those who live their lives in a chair, and one day if I am one of those people, I intend to continue to live my life to the fullest and to inspire others to do the same. None of us knows what the future may bring and what life changes we will need to accept, but I do know that experience taught me how important staying positive is and how harmful negativity can be. I fought that negative power of intention by voicing my intention to get well and keep walking. I look forward to sharing positive thoughts with other people who have MS and other diseases so that they too can learn the power of intention versus the doom of negativity.

Life and death is indeed in the power of the tongue. Let your words and thoughts be life-giving.

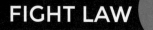

FIGHT LAW 9

EVERY TIME YOUR OPPOSITION HITS YOU, MAKE SURE YOU HIT BACK THREE TIMES AS HARD.

YOUR DETERMINATION will diminish your opposition's will to throw the same punch, and, by pure logic, it ensures that you will gain an advantage with every blow you are hit with.

With health issues, dig deep when times get rough, because the results will give you great strength. Hit the books, change up your diet, and experiment. Keep a food diary along the way. Also, believe in your body's ability to heal.

FIGHT LAW 10

PERCEPTION
IS REALITY.

REGARDLESS OF THE TRUTH, unless you are on the floor, staggering, or gasping for air, your opposition's perception of your condition is their reality. This also goes for onlookers. No one will know if you have a broken hand or rib unless you show them. The worst thing you can do is let your opposition know where and when they should attack.

As Mary discovered, one of the major issues with MS patients is that, especially in the beginning, you don't look sick, so people assume you are not. Because you don't appear to be struggling, you must not be. But this is a misguided way of thinking. In reality, everyone struggles with something each and every day.

No matter your feelings, ailments, or doubts, you must commit to a confident and capable appearance. This can cause your opponents to abandon their tactics. Most importantly, this will prevent your opposition from gaining the confidence to turn up their intensity.

In dealing with health and wellness issues, those who seek guidance through an illness need a positive approach, which is the key to wellness. Even on those days that Mary does not feel 100 percent, she tries very hard to put a smile on her face, and when asked how she is, she responds, "Great!" That statement always makes her feel better.

A positive attitude will also win the support of those around you, which will actually boost your confidence and drain that of your opposition.

CHAPTER 12

●

THE REWARD

"Why not go out on a limb?
It's where the fruit is."

●

Will Rogers

FIGHT FACT

● ●

HEALTH IS WEALTH . . .
FOR WITHOUT IT YOU HAVE LITTLE!
—Jim Coghlin Sr, Founder & Chief Volunteer, 15-40 Connection (15-40.org)

Good health is a reward in itself, but as I sat next to my daughters on the beach in Mexico recently, I was struck with a profound appreciation of my journey, the rewards of taking a risk, and the power of believing in myself.

As I sat, feeling the warmth on my face and hearing the gentle breeze blowing through the palms, making them sound as if it were raining in the sunshine, I appreciated this wonderful blessing in my life. I watched my daughters, now both young women, become friends and form an even stronger bond as sisters. My heart was filled with peace and gratitude for this wonderful week.

Just five years earlier, my pain and discomfort would have made this trip difficult, if not entirely impossible. Now we have a memory that we will cherish all of our lives. All the laughter, hugs, girl talk, and love we shared in those seven days were magical.

The power you hold within you is limitless if you truly believe that determination and faith can change the patterns of your life. I believe it is true for my life, and I believe it is for your life, too.

I thank God for the support and love of my family and friends during this difficult period of my life. Without them, my life would be drastically different.

I don't know what the future holds for me, but I do know that regardless of its challenges, I am truly blessed. And for the rest of my life, I will continue to fight to be a blessing to others.

Full Circle

On October 5, 2013, I set sail with my brothers and their wives, my nephew, and other family members for a cruise to celebrate my mother's and aunt's ninetieth and ninety-first birthdays. This cruise was such a milestone for me because the last time I had a special vacation with my mother and aunt was in 2004, when I returned home to experience a full-on medical crisis that resulted in the diagnosis of MS. Nine years later, this vacation was more than a birthday celebration; it was a testament to the miraculous changes in my life due to healthy living, and it is proof that disease can be overcome.

I am so thankful for the experiences and knowledge I have acquired over these past nine years. I am back to being a hands-on Grammy, wife, mother, sister, and friend.

Remember these three important words: Life goes on.

FIGHT LAW 11

NEVER LISTEN TO THE CROWD.

IN A FIGHT, there will be those who cheer you on, and those who jeer and try to destroy your confidence. Once again, this is a requisite of fighting and should only be regarded as confirmation that you are in the fight and have the opportunity to win something great. In Mary's case, the people at the MS golf event gave her such negative energy because she was clearly winning her fight.

Do not listen to one word from the crowd. Their vision of what is going on in the ring is rarely accurate. All they can clearly see is who gets knocked down, knocked out, and who wins and loses. The crowd can only understand the beginning and the end. They fill in the rest with hollow assumptions. They may think you are the lucky one because you are succeeding, but they may not see all the hard work that you put in to get there.

Ninety-nine percent of the crowd does not understand fighting. If they were proficient in the principles of your respective craft, they would be in the same ring themselves. And let's not forget that we are a society of quick fixes. Why hurt when you can just take a pill? Fighters look within themselves for answers.

When the fight is over, whether the crowd was cheering you on or booing, they go home, but you still have to fight another day. For a fighter, the fight never truly ends.

CHAPTER 13

THE ART OF WINNING
YOUR FIGHT

"Everybody fights, but winning is about helping others."

George Foreman III

FIGHT FACT

● ●

"FIGHT FOR THOSE THAT FIGHT FOR OTHERS. GIVE LOVE. GET LOVE."

Edwin Frias

FIGHTING MS INTO SUBMISSION was never really the end goal I was striving for when I started my fight 10 years ago. But on April 8, 2014, three weeks past the submittal date for the final copy of this book, I got some incredible news. I wanted to share with you what I wrote on that day as it truly captures my exact feelings. I thought I had won my fight by being able to walk . . . once I did that I thought I had won my fight by being able to have more energy than I did before MS . . . and then April 8th I met with my neurologist. When I got home I was so elated that I immediately wrote down my feelings.

"I went for a neurology checkup today. I went through the same testing. I felt the pin stick

I will dedicate my future to helping people believe that there is hope, to have faith in their bodies to heal, and to understand the importance of good nutrition and having a positive attitude.

into my legs, and I felt the vibration of the instrument used to test sensation and it tingled, unlike times in the past. The strength in my arms and legs was noticeable, and the doctor commented about how strong I was. I strutted down the hallway and back without hesitation and proceeded to put one foot in front of the other to make it down the hall impressively. Years earlier, there was no way I could have accomplished that feat. In the past, I needed my doctor and his assistant to hold both of my arms because I was so unsteady and might fall. I remember thinking that I would never pass a sobriety test! Then came the discussion of having another MRI. He replied, 'I don't think that it is necessary because there is no indication of deterioration.' I agreed, and he then said words that I never imagined that I would hear:

'I am classifying you as having benign multiple sclerosis. The likelihood of another relapse is remote. Whatever you are doing, keep it up. I won't need to see you again for another year. You can make the appointment now or call in a year.'"

I started this fight to beat MS. To get my life back. I have that, but I know my fight has just begun. Now my fight is to empower others, to teach and pay it forward. I never knew there was such a thing as benign MS, but I am thrilled to know there is. I will dedicate my future to helping people believe that there is hope, to have faith in their bodies to heal, and to understand the importance of good nutrition and having a positive attitude.

EVERYBODY FIGHTS! FIGHT FOR YOUR HEALTH, FIGHT TO WIN!

by George Foreman III

Join Our Fight and Tell Your Story
Everybodyfights.com/community

EVERYBODY FIGHTS, but winning is about helping others. Everybodyfights.com is a community to me. It is about building an organic community of everyday fighters. I watched my dad build his community at home one by one. I watched him fight for what he believed in, and this inspired me to go out on my own and start to make my footprint. But I wanted more than a footprint. I wanted to inspire others and build a community that thought differently from the masses. A group that is committed to helping its community; that is Type A but uses their passion, energy, and competitiveness to help those that deserve it; a group of individuals that ask themselves, "How much have I personally sacrificed to pick someone else up off the ground and help them finish their fight?"

LIVE YOUR LIFE WITH THE FIGHTING SPIRIT NEEDED TO BE AN EVERYDAY FIGHTER.

I challenge you to live your life with the Fighting Spirit needed to be an Everyday Fighter. Commit to paying it forward, and I guarantee you that it will come back around . . . but only to those that deserve it. The law of energy is one of my favorite FIGHT LAWS. Give 110%

of yourself but to the right people, to those that give you and others back 110% so that the world is not in deficit . . . this will make you better, change how we view others, and change your world.

FIGHT LAW 12

FIGHT FOR LOVE: PAY IT FORWARD.

I DID ALL MY HOMEWORK and brought my research to my dad. Watching those films taught me some invaluable lessons and gave me a new perspective on how I lived my life, but after reviewing my list, I knew something was still missing. With all the success I could ever dream up, I still didn't feel satisfied. Leave it to my dad to have the answer.

"Just give love."

Huh? He wasn't taking me seriously, and I told him so. Turns out, he was serious.

"I mean it. It's very simple, son. Name the people you love the most."

So, I listed off my parents and my siblings. Then he asked me why I love them.

Well, that's an easy answer: I just love them. They are all I've ever known. Loving my family comes naturally.

Dad asked, "Is it because they have done things to try and win your love?"

I said, "No, I just love them and they love me." He just smiled and I knew that was the right answer: Don't look for love; just give love. And then he dropped a bomb of knowledge on me in a way that only he can:

> "Love is very simple; so simple that it is nearly impossible for most to believe. You can 'make' people love you, but just as you make them love you, they can just as easily fall out of love. But when you consistently love others 'just because' —they will eventually love you back. It's a law of nature.

> "The main thing to understand is that you should not spend your years in search of love; just love others and one day you will meet someone just like yourself who is not looking for love but looking to love. You will recognize them because they are just like you. Then you will have what you are looking for."

Well said, Dad. I have to agree.

Whether you're a boxer in a ring or a person going through hardships, you have to fight for love. Great boxers fight because they love to compete, they love everything about the sport, and, of course— they love to win. They don't love the pain of battle or the agony of losing, but they use those opportunities to make them stronger, and to fuel that love.

You have to fight for love, too. Whether that's the love of a sport, the love of your job, your relationships, your health, or in loving yourself more fully, you have to fight for it, every day, through struggles and through pain. And as counterintuitive as it may seem—the best way to receive love is to give it away.

—George Foreman III

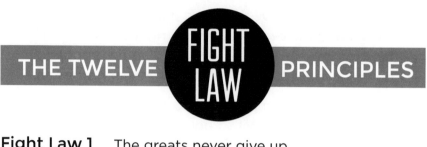

THE TWELVE FIGHT LAW PRINCIPLES

Fight Law 1 The greats never give up.

Fight Law 2 Great fighters always throw the first punch.

Fight Law 3 Goals win fights. Set them and stick to them.

Fight Law 4 Pain is the middle name of a great fighter's game.

Fight Law 5 Great fighters listen to their corner.

Fight Law 6 Greats never take a round off.

Fight Law 7 In fighting, your best defense is your offense.

Fight Law 8 When the competition is hurt or has been knocked down, great fighters do not give them the chance to recover.

Fight Law 9 Every time your opposition hits you, make sure you hit back three times as hard.

Fight Law 10 Perception is reality.

Fight Law 11 Never listen to the crowd.

Fight Law 12 Fight for love: Pay it forward.

by George Foreman III

RECIPES

EASY, HEALTHY, AND DELICIOUS

I always find it an added bonus
to read a recipe in a book like this.
It encourages the reader to begin to
prepare healthier alternatives,
especially when they realize the
healthy alternatives taste just
as good (if not better) than
foods they have been eating
for years. These recipes are some
of my favorites, and they are
also easy to prepare.

Enjoy!

●

Mary McAlary and George Foreman III

20 REASONS WHY SUGAR RUINS YOUR HEALTH

1 Sugar can suppress the immune system.

2 Sugar interferes with absorption of calcium and magnesium.

3 Sugar may make eyes more vulnerable to cataracts and age related macular degeneration.

4 Sugar can cause hypoglycemia.

5 Sugar can cause a rapid rise of adrenaline levels in children, hyperactivity, anxiety, difficulty concentrating and crankiness.

6 Sugar contributes to obesity.

7 Sugar can cause arthritis.

8 Sugar can cause heart disease and emphysema.

9 Sugar can contribute to osteoporosis.

10 Sugar can increase cholesterol.

11 Sugar can lead to several kinds of cancer including prostate, ovarian, breast cancer and more.

12 Sugar can contribute to diabetes.

13 Sugar can cause cardiovascular disease.

14 Sugar can make our skin age by changing the structure of collagen.

15 Sugar can produce a significant rise in triglycerides.

16 Sugar can increase the body's fluid retention.

17 Sugar can cause headaches, including migraines.

18 Sugar can cause depression.

19 Sugar can contribute to Alzheimer's disease.

20 Sugar contributes to the reduction in defense against bacterial infection (infectious diseases).

Above list is adapted from *146 Reasons Why Sugar Is Ruining Your Health* by Nancy Appleton, Ph.D. 2008 Integrative Nutrition 10/07

STUFFED EGGPLANTS

● ●

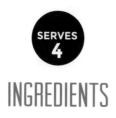

SERVES
4

INGREDIENTS

2 medium-sized eggplants

1 tbsp extra-virgin olive oil

1 small onion, chopped

2 cloves garlic, finely chopped

3/4 cup quinoa, rinse thoroughly and drain before cooking

1 1/2 cups vegetable stock

Salt and pepper to taste

2 tbsp of toasted slivered almonds

1/4 cup dried cranberries or raisins (optional)

2 tbsp of finely chopped fresh mint

1/2 cup crumbled feta cheese

Preheat the oven to 450°F. Place whole eggplants on a baking sheet and bake for approximately 15 minutes, turning once, until soft. Remove from the oven and let cool slightly.

While eggplant is in the oven, heat the olive oil in a large, heavy skillet over medium-high heat. Add the onion and garlic and cook, stirring occasionally, for about 5 minutes, or until soft. Add the rinsed quinoa, stock, salt, and pepper.

Cut each eggplant in half lengthwise and scoop out the flesh, leaving a 1/4-inch border inside the skin so that they hold their shape. Chop the flesh and stir it into the quinoa mixture in the skillet. Reduce the heat to medium-low, cover and cook for about 15 minutes, or until the quinoa is cooked through. Remove from heat and stir in the almonds, chopped mint, cranberries, and half of the cheese.

Fill the eggplant skins with the quinoa mixture and top with remaining cheese. Bake in the oven for 10–15 minutes or until the cheese is bubbling and beginning to turn brown. Garnish with mint sprigs and serve.

PORTOBELLO MUSHROOM PASTA

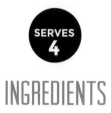

SERVES
4

INGREDIENTS

2 or 3 large Portobello mushrooms

4 quarts water

Sea salt and freshly ground black pepper

1 cup frozen shelled edamame

4 tbsp extra-virgin olive oil

2 cups of brown rice penne pasta

2 tbsp toasted sesame seeds

4 cloves of garlic, minced

2 tbsp rice wine vinegar

1 cup Roma tomatoes, chopped and drained

½ cup chopped fresh basil

½ cup chopped fresh cilantro

Remove the stalk from the mushrooms. Peel the skin off the top of the mushrooms with a small sharp knife, and then slice the mushrooms into quarter-inch slices.

In a large saucepan, bring about 4 quarts of water and a pinch of salt to a full boil. Add the frozen edamame into the boiling water and cook until the beans turn bright green. Immediately lift them out of the boiling water with a slotted spoon and transfer to a small bowl and set aside.

Into the boiling water, add 2 tablespoons of olive oil and the penne and cook until al dente. Drain the penne, but do not rinse it. Leave behind about 1 cup of the cooking water in case the pasta needs more liquid prior to serving. Put the penne back into the saucepan and cover.

Toast the sesame seeds by placing them in a small skillet and cooking until fragrant. This only takes a few minutes. Shake the pan occasionally so that they brown evenly.

In a large skillet, heat the remaining oil over medium-high heat. Add mushrooms and sauté until they become soft. Add the minced garlic and rice wine vinegar. Stir. Cover and let cook over low heat for about 5 minutes.

Place edamame in the skillet along with the tomatoes and fresh herbs. Heat through. Pour the mushroom mixture into the pot with the penne. Add sea salt and pepper to taste and add reserved pasta water, if desired. Sprinkle with toasted sesame seeds. Place pasta in a heated serving dish and serve immediately.

Sprinkle with some grated Parmesan cheese if desired.

SWISS CHARD, TOMATO, AND WHITE BEAN STEW

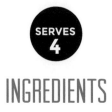

SERVES
4

INGREDIENTS

2 lbs Swiss chard, large stems discarded and leaves cut crosswise into two-inch strips

¼ cup extra-virgin olive oil

3 garlic cloves, thinly sliced

¼ tbsp crushed red pepper

1 cup canned tomatoes, chopped

1 16-oz can cannellini beans, drained and rinsed

Salt

Grated Reggiano Parmesan cheese (optional)

Bring a large saucepan of water to a boil. Add the chard and simmer over moderate heat until tender, about 8 minutes. Drain the greens and gently press out excess water.

In the saucepan, heat the oil. Add the garlic and crushed red pepper and cook over medium-low heat until the garlic is golden, about 1 minute. Be careful not to brown the garlic, as it will taste bitter. Add the tomatoes and bring to a boil. Add the beans and simmer over moderately high heat for 3 minutes. Add the chard and simmer over moderate heat until the flavors meld, about 5 minutes. Season the stew with salt and serve.

Top with some grated Parmesan cheese prior to serving.

APPLE-LEMON-GINGER JUICE WITH RAW HONEY

SERVES
1

INGREDIENTS
(all organic is best)

Throw the ½ lemon in the juicer, seeds, peel, and all. Add the ginger. Follow up with the honey (if desired) and apples cut in quarters (please remove stems and seeds).

Drink immediately to enjoy the most health benefits from the raw enzymes in the juice. As it sits, the enzymes break down. It will still be delicious, but not as healthy.

½ lemon

1 piece fresh ginger, about 1 inch long

1 tsp organic raw honey**, optional (I love Manuka honey because of its healing properties.)

2–3 apples (I prefer Granny Smith, but you can use a sweeter apple if you wish.)

NOTE: If your juicer is large enough, you may increase the ingredients for more servings.

**Do not give honey to children under two years old. They can have a serious reaction and may be too young to have built the necessary immunity.

BREAKFAST OR DESSERT YOGURT AND BERRY PARFAIT

• •

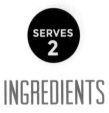

SERVES
2

INGREDIENTS

2 cups organic Greek yogurt

1/2 cup organic blueberries

1/2 cup organic raspberries

1/2 cup organic granola of your choice

Agave nectar

In two 8-ounce serving dishes, layer as follows:

1/2 of the yogurt
a layer of berries
a layer of granola

Repeat and top with granola. You can add a tablespoon of agave nectar on top for additional sweetness, if desired.

Try adding your favorite fruits and nuts to make this recipe your own.

ACKNOWLEDGMENTS

I WOULD LIKE TO EXPRESS my sincere gratitude to my family and friends who have been so supportive throughout my fight against multiple sclerosis. To my husband, Fred, for his support during the tough times; my daughter, Kristian, for her compassion and for trailblazing my way to IIN; my daughter, Marisa, for her constant care and being a great assistant in the kitchen; my son, Gaetano, for his caring and strong belief in my efforts to get well and for his introduction to my guardian angel, AJ; and my Dalai Lama, Monk, who made this book possible. To my late father, for inspiring me to fight against all odds to survive, and to my mother, whose unconditional love guides me each and every day. For all of you dog lovers, I can't forget little Marley who has become my dog and my pet therapist. She continues to watch over me, make me smile, and take me for long walks daily. Thank you to Alice Sullivan for her sensitivity and talent in putting my words on paper. To Dr. Kinkel, my sincere gratitude for the excellent care and support that you have given me over the past years. I wish you great success in your new position as Professor of Neurology, Multiple Sclerosis Division, University of California, San Diego. Many patients will benefit from your intelligence and compassion.

—**Mary McAlary**

I WOULD LIKE TO SAY my most sincere thanks to those who taught me how to fight and those who helped me get up off the canvas. To my father, George Foreman Sr., who has always been my hero and taught me through example, what fighting was all about. To my mother Andre Skeete, who taught me about survival before I knew I would ever need the skill. To my mother Mary Foreman, who taught me the value in helping others achieve their dreams. To my brother George Foreman Jr., who taught me the meaning of "mentality." To Maria Palladino Piccalo, for inspiring us with her fight swagger. To Mary, for being the inspiration we needed to publish our first book. To Bryan T. Rich, who taught me the importance of attitude, effort, and family. To Judy Rich, who taught me how important AND rewarding caring for others is. And to Anthony J. Rich, who put me back in the ring when I thought it was over.

—George Edward "Monk" Foreman III

ABOUT THE AUTHORS

MARY McALARY is an author, a realtor, a nutritionist, an organic health food specialist, a healer, a mother, and a grandmother. Mary is so many wonderful things to so many people because of one simple fact: She is a Fighter—An Everyday Fighter. Mary lives the ideology "pay it forward" every day and does so by sharing her story and sharing the knowledge she has learned on her path.

Mary McAlary was diagnosed with multiple sclerosis in 2004. She began traditional treatments, but her health continued to decline. In 2007, Mary sought out a holistic approach to battle her disease and her outcome has been remarkable. In 2008, she graduated from the Institute for Integrative Nutrition. Mary possesses a strong "Fighting Spirit," and believes that good health is attainable by organic nutrition and a healthy lifestyle. Today, her MS is benign, and she is feeling great. As a certified holistic coach, Mary enjoys sharing her knowledge for healthy living with others.

Mary McAlary lives in Andover, Massachusetts. She loves spending time with her family, cooking, and expanding her knowledge of healthy foods and lifestyles.

GEORGE FOREMAN III is a Graduate of Rice University. For the past four years George has been active as a professional boxer, achieving a record of 15-0 (14 KO's). From 2002–2009, George served as his father's, George Foreman Sr., manager. Every interview, endorsement contract, publishing agreement, television/movie contract, and marketing campaign involving George Foreman Sr. was negotiated and/or executed under the direct supervision of George III.

After over ten years in the world of sports management, marketing, and being an athlete himself, George decided to combine the knowledge and experience from the two industries he knows best to form *The Club*; a lifestyle fitness brand that embodies the concept EVERYBODYFIGHTS. Understanding the need for a truly authentic fitness community based around The Fighting Spirit, George saw an opportunity to provide a third home for the Everyday Fighter while servicing a sincere need in the market—providing a FUN fitness environment that motivates its clients inside the facility and out. *The Club* is a community driven by its members of all ages and demographics. If you are an everyday fighter and embody our fighting spirit, then you belong with us! EVERYBODYFIGHTS.

HIGHLIGHTS:

Professional Boxer 15-0 (14 KO's)

2013: Opening First Flagship Fitness Club in Boston's Seaport District

2002–2009: Business Manager for George Foreman Sr.

2008: Executive Producer for the ABC prime-time show, *American Inventor*

2007: Executive Producer of Reality TV Show *Family Foreman* on TVLAND

2006: Graduated From Rice University with a Degree in Sports Management

2006: Appeared on the E! Reality TV show, *Filthy Rich Cattle Drive*

2005: Structured deal to take George Foreman Enterprises public through a reverse merger

---